89 Juice and Salad Recipes to Fight Cancer:

The Comprehensive Recipe Book to Combating Cancer No Matter What Your Condition

By

Joe Correa CSN

COPYRIGHT

This publication is designed to provide accurate and authoritative information in regard to the subject matter covered. It is sold with the understanding that neither the author nor the publisher is engaged in rendering medical advice. If medical advice or assistance is needed, consult with a doctor. This book is considered a guide and should not be used in any way detrimental to your health. Consult with a physician before starting this nutritional plan to make sure it's right for you.

ACKNOWLEDGEMENTS

This book is dedicated to my friends and family that have had mild or serious illnesses so that you may find a solution and make the necessary changes in your life.

89 Juice and Salad Recipes to Fight Cancer:

The Comprehensive Recipe Book to Combating Cancer No Matter What Your Condition

By

Joe Correa CSN

CONTENTS

ABOUT THE AUTHOR

After years of Research, I honestly believe in the positive effects that proper nutrition can have over the body and mind. My knowledge and experience has helped me live healthier throughout the years and which I have shared with family and friends. The more you know about eating and drinking healthier, the sooner you will want to change your life and eating habits.

Nutrition is a key part in the process of being healthy and living longer so get started today. The first step is the most important and the most significant.

INTRODUCTION

89 Juice and Salad Recipes to Fight Cancer: The Comprehensive Recipe Book to Combating Cancer No Matter What Your Condition

By Joe Correa CSN

In the past couple of decades, cancer has escalated to epidemic proportions and affects nearly one out of two men and one out of three women. With 7-8 million lives taken each year due to this disease, I can definitely say that preventing cancer should be your number one priority.

One of the major causes for this disease is our modern lifestyles which surround us with different toxins, cancerous substances, and stress. But the main reason is probably poor nutrition for most people. The lack of basic nutrients weakens our immune system which leads to serious and long-term damage to your health and eventually becomes cancer. Most food is full of artificial flavors, colors, additives, stabilizers, and preservatives. Although some of these substances are harmless, many of them are extremely toxic and can deprive our organism of some important nutrients. Although most people know these facts, in theory, they can't seem to find enough time to plan their meals on a daily basis, which is why fast food has become so popular.

These cancer preventing recipes are designed to give you exactly that, all the important nutrients in just a couple of minutes. Try them and see what a difference they can make in your life and the life of your loved ones!

COMMITMENT

In order to improve my condition, I *(your name)*, commit to eating more of these foods on a daily basis and to exercise at least 30 minutes daily:

-   Berries (especially blueberries), peaches, cherries, apples, apricots, oranges, lemon juice, grapefruit, tangerines, mandarins, pears, etc.
-   Broccoli, spinach, collard greens, sweet potatoes, avocado, artichoke, baby corn, carrots, celery, cauliflower, onions, etc.
-   Whole grains, steel-cut oats, oatmeal, quinoa, barley, etc.
-   Black beans, red bean beans, garbanzo beans, lentils, etc.
-   Nuts and seeds including: walnuts, cashews, flaxseeds, sesame seeds, etc.
-   Fish
-   8 – 10 glasses of water

Sign here

X_____

89 JUICE AND SALAD RECIPES TO FIGHT CANCER: THE COMPREHENSIVE RECIPE BOOK TO COMBATING CANCER NO MATTER WHAT YOUR CONDITION

1. Sweet Potato Carrot Juice

Ingredients:

2 large carrots

1 small sweet potato, peeled

2 medium-sized green apples, cored

1 large orange, peeled

¼ tsp of pumpkin pie spice

Preparation:

Combine all ingredients except pumpkin pie spice in a juicer and process until juiced.

Transfer the juice to serving glasses and add few ice cubes.

Sprinkle with some pumpkin pie spice and serve.

Nutritional information per serving: Kcal: 147, Protein: 2.1g, Carbs: 35.4g, Fats: 0.1g

2.   Ginger Chia Juice

Ingredients:

3 large carrots

2 large apples, cored

½ tsp of ginger, ground

1 tbsp of chia seeds

Preparation:

Combine all ingredients except chia seeds in a juicer and process until juiced.

Transfer to serving glasses and add few ice cubes. Sprinkle with chia seeds before serving for extra nutrients. Enjoy!

Nutritional information per serving: Kcal: 177, Protein: 3.2g, Carbs: 28.4g, Fats: 4.6g

3. Kale Squash Juice

Ingredients:

¼ cup of fresh kale

½ yellow squash, peeled

1 medium-sized broccoli

1 large apple, cored

¼ cup of fresh spinach

4 small carrots

Preparation:

Combine all ingredients in a juicer and process until juiced.

Transfer to serving glasses and add few ice cubes. Serve immediately.

Nutritional information per serving: Kcal: 81, Protein: 2.3g, Carbs: 18.4g, Fats: 0.2g

4.   Watermelon Juice

Ingredients:

1 cup of watermelon, peeled and seeded

1 cup of pineapple, peeled

½ large lemon, peeled

½ tsp of ginger, ground

Preparation:

Combine all ingredients in a juicer and process until juiced.

Transfer to serving glasses and add few ice cubes. Serve immediately!

Nutritional information per serving: Kcal: 41, Protein: 1.4g, Carbs: 10.2g, Fats: 0.1g

5.   Cancun Juice

Ingredients:

½ cup of fresh kale

1 large lime, peeled

1 large cucumber

1 celery stalk

1 small jalapeno pepper, seeded

Preparation:

Combine all ingredients in a juicer and process until juiced. Add coconut water if it is too spicy.

Transfer to serving glasses and add a few ice cubes.

Serve immediately.

Nutritional information per serving: Kcal: 171, Protein: 3.2g, Carbs: 47.3g, Fats: 1.3g

6.   Flaxseed Brown Juice

Ingredients:

2 large carrots

½ cup of fresh spinach

2 tbsp of fresh parsley

2 large apples, cored

¼ tsp of ginger, ground

1 tbsp of flaxseeds

Preparation:

Combine all ingredients in a juicer except flaxseeds. Process until juiced.

Transfer to serving glasses and add few ice cubes.

Sprinkle with flaxseeds and serve!

Nutritional information per serving: Kcal: 119, Protein: 4.3g, Carbs: 62.2g, Fats: 2.3g

7.   Lemon Kale Juice

Ingredients:

½ cup of fresh kale

1 lemon, peeled

2 large green apples, cored

1 large pear, cored

Preparation:

Combine all ingredients in a juicer and process until juiced.

Transfer to serving glasses and add few ice cubes before serving.

Enjoy!

Nutritional information per serving: Kcal: 120, Protein: 3.2g, Carbs: 62.5g, Fats: 1.2g

8.   Broccoli Juice

Ingredients:

1 cup of broccoli

2 large oranges, peeled

1 large cucumber, peeled

1 large carrot

Preparation:

Combine all ingredients in a juicer and process until juiced.

Transfer to serving glasses and add few ice cubes.

Serve immediately!

Nutritional information per serving: Kcal: 68, Protein: 2.3g, Carbs: 19.7g, Fats: 0.1g

9.   Collard Green Juice

Ingredients:

½ cup of collard greens

½ tsp of ginger, ground

1 large cucumber

¼ cup of fresh parsley

1 large apple, cored

Preparation:

Combine all ingredients in a juicer and process until juiced.

Transfer to serving glasses and add few ice cubes.

Serve immediately.

Nutritional information per serving: Kcal: 96, Protein: 3.1g, Carbs: 28.7g, Fats: 1.2g

10.   Fennel Tangerine Juice

Ingredients:

1 large fennel

½ cup of fresh kale

1 large green apple, cored

4 tangerines, peeled

Preparation:

Place all ingredients in a juicer and process until juiced.

Transfer to serving glasses and add few ice cubes or refrigerate before use.

Nutritional information per serving: Kcal: 121, Protein: 4.3g, Carbs: 31.3g, Fats: 1.3g

11.   Green Grape Juice

Ingredients:

1 cup of green grapes

2 large cucumbers

1 large pear, cored

1 lime, peeled

Preparation:

Combine all ingredients in a juicer and process until juiced.

Transfer to serving glasses and refrigerate for 30 minutes before serving.

Nutritional information per serving: Kcal: 113, Protein: 18.3g, Carbs: 31.3g, Fats: 0.1g

12.   Watercress Juice

Ingredients:

½ cup of watercress

2 large green apples, cored

1 large lemon, peeled

1 large lime, peeled

Preparation:

Combine all ingredients except chia seeds in a juicer and process until juiced.

Transfer to serving glasses and add few ice cubes.

Serve immediately.

Nutritional information per serving: Kcal: 101, Protein: 17.2g, Carbs: 28.8g, Fats: 0.2g

13.   Pineapple Cantaloupe Juice

Ingredients:

1 cup of cantaloupe, peeled

½ pineapple, peeled

2 large green apples, cored

½ cup of fresh kale

Preparation:

Combine all ingredients in a juicer and process until juiced.

Transfer to serving glasses and add few ice cubes, or refrigerate for 30 minutes before serving.

Nutritional information per serving: Kcal: 115, Protein: 1.2g, Carbs: 28.8g, Fats: 1.2g

14.   Radish Fennel Juice

Ingredients:

6 medium-sized radishes

1 small fennel

1 large orange, peeled

5 large celery stalks

1 large cucumber

Preparation:

Combine all ingredients in a juicer and process until juiced.

Transfer to serving glasses and refrigerate for a while before serving.

Nutritional information per serving: Kcal: 110, Protein: 6.1g, Carbs: 28.7g, Fats: 1.2g

15.   Swiss Chard Basil Juice

Ingredients:

½ cup of Swiss chard

½ cup of fresh basil

1 large lime, peeled

2 large green apples, cored

¼ cup of fresh mint

Preparation:

Combine all ingredients in a juicer and process until juiced.

Transfer to serving glasses and add few ice cubes or refrigerate until use.

Nutritional information per serving: Kcal: 114, Protein: 2.3g, Carbs: 30.4g, Fats: 0.2g

16.   Green Cabbage Juice

Ingredients:

½ cup of green cabbage

4 celery stalks

1 large green apple, cored

3 large carrots

1 large lemon, peeled

1 tbsp of liquid honey

Preparation:

Combine all ingredients in a juicer and process until juiced.

Transfer to serving glasses and refrigerate for 20 minutes before serving.

Nutritional information per serving: Kcal: 162, Protein: 3.1g, Carbs: 39.3g, Fats: 0.1g

17.   Grapefruit Rosemary Juice

Ingredients:

3 large grapefruits, peeled

3 large oranges, peeled

1 large lemon, peeled

½ tsp of fresh rosemary

Preparation:

Combine all ingredients in a juicer and process until juiced.

Transfer to serving glasses and add few ice cubes.

Sprinkle with fresh rosemary and serve immediately!

Nutritional information per serving: Kcal: 140, Protein: 3.4g, Carbs: 37.6g, Fats: 0.1g

18.   Strawberry Peach Juice

Ingredients:

3 large peaches, pitted

1 cup of strawberries

1 large green apple, cored

¼ tsp of ginger, ground

Preparation:

Combine all ingredients in a juicer and process until juiced.

Transfer to serving glasses and add few ice cubes, or refrigerate for 1 hour before serving.

Nutritional information per serving: Kcal: 64, Protein: 1.2g, Carbs: 18.3g, Fats: 0.1g

19.   Cilantro Juice

Ingredients:

½ cup of cilantro

3 celery stalks

1 large green apple, cored

1 large lemon, peeled

½ tsp of ginger, ground

Preparation:

Combine all ingredients except ginger in a juicer.

Process until juiced and transfer to serving glasses and stir in the ginger.

Add few ice cubes and serve immediately.

Nutritional information per serving: Kcal: 73, Protein: 2.2g, Carbs: 26.7g, Fats: 0.1g

20. Pomegranate Kale Juice

Ingredients:

½ cup of pomegranate seeds

½ cup of fresh kale

1 large green apple, cored

¼ tsp of ginger, ground

3-4 fresh mint leaves

Preparation:

Combine pomegranate seeds, kale, mint, and apple in a juicer and process until juiced.

Transfer to serving glasses and stir in the ginger and some extra pomegranate seeds if you like.

Add few ice cubes and serve immediately.

Nutritional information per serving: Kcal: 143, Protein: 6.2g, Carbs: 41.2g, Fats: 2.4g

21.   Tomato Garlic Juice

Ingredients:

2 large tomatoes, halved

2 garlic cloves, peeled

3 large cucumbers

1 large bell pepper, seeded

1 small shallot

1 large lime, peeled

¼ cup of fresh cilantro

Preparation:

Combine all ingredients in a juicer and process until juiced.

Transfer to serving glasses and add few ice cubes or refrigerate for a while before serving.

Nutritional information per serving: Kcal: 109, Protein: 6.4g, Carbs: 38.5g, Fats: 1.2g

22. Pineapple Carrot Juice

Ingredients:

1 cup of pineapple, peeled

2 large carrots

½ cup of watercress

1 large lemon, peeled

¼ tsp of ginger root

Preparation:

Combine all ingredients in a juicer and process until juiced.

Transfer to serving glasses and enjoy!

Nutritional information per serving: Kcal: 101, Protein: 3.1g, Carbs: 34.2g, Fats: 1.1g

23.   Strawberry Kiwi Juice

Ingredients:

2 kiwis, peeled

1 large cucumber

1 cup of fresh strawberries

1 small lime, peeled

2 tbsp of fresh mint

Preparation:

Combine all ingredients in a juicer and process until juiced.

Transfer to serving glasses and refrigerate for a while until use.

Nutritional information per serving: Kcal: 91, Protein: 3.1g, Carbs: 29.9g, Fats: 0.9g

24.   Apple Chia Juice

Ingredients:

1 large red apple, cored

1 large lemon, peeled

1 large bell pepper, seeded

3 tbsp of chia seeds

Preparation:

Combine apple, lemon, and bell pepper and run trough juicer.

Process until juiced and stir in the chia seeds.

Let it stand for 15 minutes to thicken and stir well before use.

Nutritional information per serving: Kcal: 135, Protein: 4.2g, Carbs: 31.3g, Fats: 6.2g

25.   Spicy Grapefruit Juice

Ingredients:

1 large kiwi, peeled

½ medium-sized grapefruit, peeled

1 large lemon, peeled

3 celery stalks

¼ tsp of ginger, ground

¼ tsp of Cayenne pepper, ground

A handful of watercress

Preparation:

Combine kiwi, grapefruit, lemon, celery, and watercress in a juicer and process until juiced.

Transfer to serving glasses and stir in the ginger and cayenne pepper.

Enjoy!

Nutritional information per serving: Kcal: 61, Protein: 2.1g, Carbs: 20.4g, Fats: 1.1g

26.   Turmeric Cucumber Juice

Ingredients:

1 large cucumber

1 cup of pineapple, chopped

3 celery stalks

½ cup of fresh spinach

¼ tsp of ginger, ground

¼ tsp of turmeric, ground

Preparation:

Combine all ingredients except ginger and turmeric in a juicer.

Process until juiced and transfer to serving glasses. Stir in the turmeric and ginger and serve.

Nutritional information per serving: Kcal: 109, Protein: 3.3g, Carbs: 61.2g, Fats: 1.3g

27.   Zucchini Roma Juice

Ingredients:

2 medium-sized zucchini

1 garlic clove, peeled

6 asparagus stalks

3 Roma tomatoes

4 large carrots

Preparation:

Combine all ingredients in a juicer and process until juiced.

Transfer to serving glasses and enjoy immediately.

Nutritional information per serving: Kcal: 92, Protein: 5.4g, Carbs: 27.3g, Fats: 0.9g

28.   Cinnamon Chia Juice

Ingredients:

1 tbsp of chia seeds

1 large apple, cored

1 cup of fresh spinach

¼ tsp of cinnamon, ground

Preparation:

Combine apple and spinach in a juicer and process until juiced.

Transfer to serving glasses and stir in the cinnamon and chia seeds.

Set aside for 20 minutes to thicken, then serve.

Nutritional information per serving: Kcal: 121, Protein: 4.3g, Carbs: 27.8g, Fats: 5.3g

29.   Green Coconut Juice

Ingredients:

1 large lime, peeled

3 oz of coconut water

5 small celery stalks

¼ cup od fresh mint

¼ cup of fresh spinach

Preparation:

Combine lime, celery, spinach, and mint in a juicer and process until juiced.

Transfer to serving glasses and stir in coconut water. Refrigerate for 20 minutes before use.

Nutritional information per serving: Kcal: 45, Protein: 2.2g, Carbs: 16.8g, Fats: 1.6g

30.   Cauliflower Broccoli Juice

Ingredients:

2 cups of cauliflower, chopped

1 cup of fresh broccoli

4 large carrots

1 large green apple, cored

1 tsp of ginger root

Preparation:

Combine all ingredients in a juicer and process until juiced.

Transfer to serving glasses and garnish with mint or add ice cubes for refreshment.

Enjoy!

Nutritional information per serving: Kcal: 136, Protein: 6.3g, Carbs: 42.8g, Fats: 1.2g

31. Ice Green Juice

Ingredients:

1 medium-sized cucumber

1 large pear, cored

3 large carrots

1 large lemon, peeled

¼ cup of fresh mint

½ cup of broccoli

1 tsp of ginger root

½ tsp of green tea powder

2 oz of water

Preparation:

Combine cucumber, pear, carrots, lemon, mint, ginger, and broccoli in a juicer and process until juiced. Mix water with green tea in a serving glasses and add juice. Mix with a spoon and add few ice cubes. Serve immediately.

Nutritional information per serving: Kcal: 141, Protein: 5.5g, Carbs: 45.7g, Fats: 0.9g

32. Orange Green Juice

Ingredients:

2 large oranges, peeled

½ cup of fresh broccoli, chopped

3 large carrots

4 collard green leaves

4 fresh kale leaves

1 garlic clove, peeled

Preparation:

Combine all ingredients in a juicer and process until juiced.

Transfer to serving glasses and serve immediately.

Nutritional information per serving: Kcal: 171, Protein: 9.2g, Carbs: 43.3g, Fats: 2.3g

33.   Orange Honey Juice

Ingredients:

2 large oranges, peeled

½ cup of grapefruit, chopped

3-4 fresh kale leaves

1 tsp of liquid honey

¼ tsp of ginger, ground

Preparation:

Combine oranges, grapefruit, and kale in a juicer and process until juiced.

Transfer to serving glasses and stir in the honey and ginger.

Serve immediately.

Nutritional information per serving: Kcal: 128, Protein: 7.3g, Carbs: 34.5g, Fats: 1.1g

34.   Sweet Potato Ginger Juice

Ingredients:

2 medium-sized sweet potatoes, peeled

1 large peach, pitted and halved

¼ tsp of ginger, ground

¼ tsp of cinnamon, ground

Preparation:

Combine potatoes and peach in a juicer and process until juiced.

Transfer to serving glasses and stir in the ginger and cinnamon.

Serve immediately.

Nutritional information per serving: Kcal: 159, Protein: 5.2g, Carbs: 50.1g, Fats: 0.9g

35.   Strawberry Tomato Juice

Ingredients:

1 cup of fresh strawberries

2 large tomatoes

2 large carrots

1 large orange, peeled

1 large bell pepper, seeded

Preparation:

Combine all ingredients in a juicer and process until juiced.

Transfer to serving glasses and refrigerate for 30 minutes before serving.

Nutritional information per serving: Kcal: 104, Protein: 3.9g, Carbs: 31.2g, Fats: 1.1g

36.   Orange Turmeric Juice

Ingredients:

1 large orange bell pepper, seeded

1 large orange, peeled

1 large carrot

1 large lemon, peeled

1 small cucumber

¼ tsp of turmeric, ground

Preparation:

Combine all ingredients except turmeric in a juicer and process until juiced.

Transfer to serving glasses and stir in the turmeric. Serve immediately.

Nutritional information per serving: Kcal: 152, Protein: 4.2g, Carbs: 48.1g, Fats: 1.3g

37.   Arugula Juice

Ingredients:

1 cup of fresh arugula

1 large lemon, peeled

1 large lime, peeled

1 large orange, peeled

1 large kiwi, peeled

1 small cucumber

Preparation:

Combine all ingredients in a juicer and process until juiced.

Transfer to serving glasses and serve immediately.

Nutritional information per serving: Kcal: 192, Protein: 3.1g, Carbs: 31.6g, Fats: 0.9g

38.   Mango Juice

Ingredients:

1 large mango, peeled

1 large cucumber

½ cup of fresh spinach

2 oz of coconut, grated

Preparation:

Combine mango, cucumber, and spinach in a juicer and process until juiced.

Transfer to serving glasses and stir in the grated coconut.

Refrigerate for 1 hour before serving.

Nutritional information per serving: Kcal: 68, Protein: 1.9g, Carbs: 20.1g, Fats: 0.5g

39.   Bok Choy Leek Juice

Ingredients:

1 medium-sized leek

1 small baby bok choy

¼ cup of fresh basil

1 large green apple, cored

2 large carrots

4-5 fresh kale leaves

Preparation:

Combine all ingredients in a juicer and process until juiced.

Transfer to serving glasses and refrigerate before use.

Nutritional information per serving: Kcal: 169, Protein: 2.3g, Carbs: 46.2g, Fats: 1.9g

40.   Strawberry Kale Juice

Ingredients:

2 cups of fresh strawberries

1 large green apple, cored

1 large cucumber

4-5 fresh kale leaves

Preparation:

Combine all ingredients in a juicer and process until juiced.

Transfer to serving glasses and serve immediately.

Nutritional information per serving: Kcal: 184, Protein: 7.7g, Carbs: 49.5g, Fats: 2.1g

SALAD RECIPES

1.   Strawberry Spinach Salad

Ingredients:

4 oz strawberries, chopped

4 oz grapes

1 large cucumber, chunked

1 small red bell pepper, chopped

1 tbsp olive oil

½ whole lime, juiced

2 cups fresh spinach, chopped

1 tbsp sunflower seeds

1 tbsp fresh basil, chopped

Salt to taste

Preparation:

Rinse the strawberries under running water and drain. Remove the stems and chop into bite-sized pieces. Set aside.

Wash the cucumber and cut into small chunks. Set aside.

Wash the pepper and cut lengthwise in half. Remove the stem and seeds. Chop into small pieces and set aside.

In a small mixing bowl, combine olive oil, lime juice, and salt. Mix until combined and set aside.

Now, combine spinach, strawberries, grapes, cucumber, and red bell pepper in a large salad bowl. Drizzle with previously prepared dressing and top with sunflower seeds and basil.

Serve immediately.

Nutritional information per serving: Kcal: 347, Protein: 7g, Carbs: 50.9g, Fats: 17.1g

2.   Spanish Tuna Steak Salad

Ingredients:

4 oz tuna steaks

2 medium-sized tomatoes, chopped

1 large cucumber, sliced

1 medium-sized purple onion, sliced

¼ cup green olives, pitted

2 eggs, hard-boiled

1 whole lime, sliced

2 tbsp olive oil

2 tsp red wine vinegar

½ tsp dried rosemary, ground

½ tsp dried thyme, ground

Salt and pepper to taste

Preparation:

Rinse the meat under running water and pat-dry with a kitchen paper. Transfer to a cutting board and cut into thin slices.

Preheat 1 tasblespoon of oil in a skillet over medium-high heat. Add tuna steaks and sprinkle with salt, pepper, thyme, and rosemary. Cook for 2-3 minutes on each side. Remove from the heat and set aside.

Place the egg in a deep pot and add water enough to cover. Bring to a boil and then cook for 10-13 minutes. Remove from the heat and transfer to a bowl with ice cold water. When chilled, peel and chop into small pieces.

Wash and prepare the vegetables.

In a small mixing bowl, combine the remaining olive oil, red wine vinegar, dried rosemary, dried thyme, salt, and pepper. Mix until combined and set aside.

Now, combine tomatoes, cucumber, purple onion, olives, and eggs in a large salad bowl. Drizzle with previously prepared dressing and top with tuna steaks.

Serve immediately.

Nutritional information per serving: Kcal: 347, Protein: 7g, Carbs: 50.9g, Fats: 17.1g

3. **Broccoli Kale Salad**

Ingredients:

2 cups broccoli, chopped

2 cups fresh kale, chopped

1 small onion, chopped

1 small cucumber, sliced

½ cup cherry tomatoes, halved

1 tbsp extra-virgin olive oil

½ tsp dried oregano, ground

½ tsp dried thyme, ground

½ tsp salt

¼ tsp black pepper, ground

Preparation:

Rinse the broccoli under cold running water and drain. Cut into bite-sized pieces and transfer to a large pot. Add water enough to cover and bring to a boil over medium-high heat. Cook for 5 minutes and remove from the heat. Drain well and set aside.

In a small bowl, combine olive oil, dried oregano, dried thyme, salt, and pepper. Mix until well combined and set aside.

Wash and prepare the remaining ingredients.

Now, combine kale, cherry tomatoes, onion, cucumber, and cooked broccoli in a large salad bowl. Drizzle with the dressing and serve.

Optionally, sprinkle all with some lemon or lime juice for some extra flavor.

Enjoy!

Nutritional information per serving: Kcal: 342, Protein: 12.8g, Carbs: 48.2g, Fats: 15.3g

4. Tomato Onion Salad with Citrus Dressing

Ingredients:

1 cup cherry tomatoes, halved

1 small cucumber, sliced

¼ cup Feta cheese, crumbled

1 small purple onion, chopped

5 green olives, pitted and chopped

1 whole lemon, juiced

2 tbsp orange juice, freshly squeezed

2 tbsp extra-virgin olive oil

1 tbsp balsamic vinegar

½ tsp dried oregano, ground

Salt and pepper to taste

Preparation:

In a small mixing bowl, combine lemon juice, orange juice, olive oil, balsamic vinegar, dried oregano, salt, and pepper. Mix until well combined and set aside.

Rinse the cherry tomatoes under running water and

remove the stems. Cut into halves and transfer to a large bowl.

Wash the cucumber and cut into thin slices. Add to the bowl and set aside.

Peel the onion and chop into small pieces. Transfer to a small colander and rinse under water. Transfer to the bowl with the remaining vegetables.

Add crumbled cheese and drizzle with previously prepared dressing. Mix until well combined and serve immediately.

Enjoy!

Nutritional information per serving: Kcal: 249, Protein: 5.2g, Carbs: 16.1g, Fats: 19.9g

5.   **Mango Berry Salad**

Ingredients:

1 large mango, chopped

½ cup fresh strawberries, chopped

½ cup fresh blueberries

½ cup fresh raspberries

1 cup grapes

1 medium-sized apple, chopped

1 large orange, peeled and wedged

3 tbsp fresh orange juice

1 tsp lemon zest, freshly grated

2 tsp liquid stevia

Preparation:

Peel the mango and remove the pit. Chop into bite-sized pieces and set aside.

In a large colander, combine strawberries, blueberries, and raspberries. Rinse under running water and drain. Remove the stems from the strawberries and chop into bite-sized pieces.

Wash the apple and cut lengthwise in half. Remove the core and cut into small pieces.

Peel the orange and divide into wedges. Cut each wedge in half and set aside.

In a small mixing bolw, combine orange juice, lemon zest, and stevia. Mix until combined and set aside.

Mix fruit in a large salad bowl and drizzle with previously prepared dressing. Toss to combine and chil in the refrigerator for 20 minutes before serving.

Enjoy!

Nutritional information per serving: Kcal: 292, Protein: 3.9g, Carbs: 73.6g, Fats: 1.6g

6.   Asparagus Dijon Salad

Ingredients:

10 oz fresh asparagus, trimmed and chopped

½ cup cherry tomatoes, chopped

¼ cup ricotta cheese, crumbled

1 tbsp walnuts, finely chopped

1 garlic clove, finely chopped

1 tbsp olive oil

2 tbsp balsamic vinegar

2 tsp Dijon mustard

Salt and pepper to taste

Preparation:

Rinse the asparagus under running water and drain. Transfer to a cutting board and trim off the woody ends. Chop into bite-sized pieces and transfer to a deep pot. Add water enough to cover and bring to a boil over medium-high heat. Cook for 3 minutes and remove from the heat. Drain and set aside.

Wash the tomatoes and trim off the stems. Chop into small

pieces and set aside.

In a small mixing bowl, combine finely chopped garlic, olive oil, balsamic vinegar, Dijon mustard, salt, and pepper. Mix until well combined.

In a large salad bowl, combine asparagus, tomatoes, and ricotta cheese. Drizzle with previously prepared dressing. Sprinkle with walnuts and toss until combined.

Serve immediately.

Nutritional information per serving: Kcal: 344, Protein: 16.6g, Carbs: 20.3g, Fats: 24.4g

7.   Pineapple Chicken Salad

Ingredients:

1 cup pineapple, chunked

6 oz chicken breast, skinless and boneless

2 cups fresh baby spinach

1 small purple onion, chopped

¼ cup Mozzarella cheese, sliced

2 tbsp avocado oil

2 tbsp cider vinegar

1 garlic clove, minced

¼ tsp cayenne pepper

Salt

Preparation:

Rinse the chicken under running water and pat-dry with a kitchen paper. Transfer to a cutting board and cut into bite-sized pieces. Transfer to a bowl and sprinkle with salt and cayenne pepper. Mix well with your hands and set aside.

Preheat one tablespoon of avocado oil in a skillet over

medium-high heat. Add chicken and cook for 5 minutes, stirring ocassionally. Remove from the heat and set aside.

Using a sharp knife, remove the top of a pineapple. Carefully peel and cut into 1-inch thick rings. Now, chop into bite-sized pieces and fill the measuring cup. Reserve the rest in the refrigerator.

Rinse the spinach under running water. Drain and transfer to a large salad bowl. Add pineapple, chopped onion, and cheese.

In a small mixing bowl, combine the remaining avocado oil, vinegar, and minced garlic. Mix until combined and drizzle over the salad. Stir once and top with chicken.

Serve immediately.

Nutritional information per serving: Kcal: 194, Protein: 21g, Carbs: 16.9g, Fats: 4.9g

8.   Watermelon Cheese Salad

Ingredients:

4 cups watermelon, cut into chunks

1 cup Mozzarella cheese, sliced

1 cup baby spinach

1 tbsp fresh basil, finely chopped

½ tsp sea salt

½ tsp black pepper, ground

2 tbsp extra-virgin olive oil

1 tsp balsamic vinegar

Preparation:

Cut the watermelon in half. Cut and peel 3-4 large wedges. Chop into small chunks and remove the pits. Fill the measuring cups and reserve the rest in the refrigerator.

Rinse the baby spinach under running water using a colander. Drain and place in a large salad bowl.

Add watermelon chunks to the bowl along with mozzarella cheese. Sprinkle with salt, pepper, and basil.

Drizzle with olive oil and balsamic vinegar. Toss to combine and serve immediately.

Nutritional information per serving: Kcal: 257, Protein: 6.3g, Carbs: 24.3g, Fats: 17g

9.   Broccoli Carrot Salad with Almonds

Ingredients:

3 cups broccoli, chopped

2 large carrots, shredded

½ small red onion, chopped

2 tbsp dried cranberries

2 tbsp almonds, roughly chopped

2 tbsp lemon juice, freshly squeezed

Salt and pepper to taste

Preparation:

Rinse the broccoli under running water using a large colander. Drain and chop into bite-sized pieces. Transfer to a large saucepan and cover with water. Add a pinch of salt and bring to a boil over medium-high heat. Cook for 2-3 minutes. Remove from the heat and transfer to a colander using a slotted spoon. Rinse under cold water and set aside.

Wash and prepare the remaining vegetables.

Now, in a large salad bowl, combine broccoli, carrots, and onion. Drizzle with fresh lemon juice and stir until combined.

Top with cranberries and almonds and serve immediately.

Nutritional information per serving: Kcal: 250, Protein: 12g, Carbs: 40g, Fats: 7.1g

10.   Bean Avocado Salad

Ingredients:

1 cup black beans, soaked overnight

1 large bell pepper, chopped

½ ripe avocado, sliced

1 small onion, chopped

1 tbsp extra-virgin olive oil

1 whole lime, juiced

¼ tsp cumin powder

1 tbsp spring onions, chopped

¼ tsp cayenne pepper, ground

Preparation:

Drain the beans and rinse under running water. Transfer to a deep pot and cover with 2 cups of water. Bring to a boil over medium-high heat. Cook for 20-25 minutes. Remove from the heat and drain well. Set aside.

Cut the bell pepper in half. Remove the stem and seeds. Rinse once and chop into bite-sized pieces. Set aside.

Peel the avocado and cut in half. Remove the pit and cut one half into bite-sized pieces. Reserve the rest in the refrigerator.

In a large salad bowl, combine beans, bell pepper, avocado, and chopped onion. Sprinkle with olive oil, lime juice, cumin powder, and cayenne pepper. Stir until well combined and sprinkle with spring onions before serving.

Nutritional information per serving: Kcal: 353, Protein: 15.4g, Carbs: 48.7g, Fats: 12.3g

11.   Quinoa Tomato Salad

Ingredients:

1 cup quinoa

2 cups cherry tomatoes, chopped

1 medium-sized cucumber, sliced

1 small red onion, chopped

¼ cup cottage cheese, crumbled

1 tbsp fresh parsley, finely chopped

2 tbsp extra-virgin olive oil

2 tsp red wine vinegar

½ tsp garlic powder

½ tsp smoked paprika, ground

½ tsp dried oregano, ground

Salt and pepper to taste

Preparation:

Place the quinoa in a large colander and rinse under running water. Drain and transfer to a heavy-bottomed pot. Add 2 cups of water and bring to a boil over medium-high heat. Reduce the heat to low and simmer for 10-15 minutes, or until all the liquid has been absorbed. Remove from the heat and fluff with a fork.

In a mixing bowl, combine olive oil, red wine vinegar, garlic powder, smoked paprika, oregano, salt, and pepper. Mix until well incorporated and set aside.

In a large salad bowl, combine quinoa, tomatoes, cucumber, and onion. Drizzle with previously prepared dressing and toss to combine.

Serve immediately.

Nutritional information per serving: Kcal: 267, Protein: 9.6g, Carbs: 36.2g, Fats: 10.2g

12.   Shrimp Potato Salad

Ingredients:

6 oz shrimps, cleaned and deveined

2 medium-sized potatoes, chopped

1 medium-sized tomato, chopped

1 small onion, sliced

1 garlic clove, minced

2 tbsp olive oil

½ whole lime, juiced

1 tbsp fresh cilantro, finely chopped

1 tsp Dijon mustard

Salt and pepper to taste

Preparation:

In a small mixing bowl, combine garlic, olive oil, lime juice, cilantro, Dijon mustard, salt, and pepper. Mix until combined and set aside.

Pour 3 cups of water in a deep pot. Bring to a boil over medium-high heat. Place the shrimps in a steam basked and place on top of the pot. Make sure that the shrimps are not submerged. Sprinkle with some salt and steam for 10 minutes, or until pink. Remove the basket from the pot and set aside.

Peel the potatoes and cut into small chunks. Rinse and transfer to a heavy-bottomed pot. Add water enough to cover and bring to a boil over medium-high heat. Cook until fork-tender and remove from the heat. Drain and set aside.

Now, combine potatoes, tomato, and onion in a large salad bowl. Top with shrimps and drizzle with previously prepared dressing.

Serve cold.

Nutritional information per serving: Kcal: 265, Protein: 16.1g, Carbs: 27.4g, Fats: 10.6g

13.   Steamed Salmon Caprese Salad

Ingredients:

6 oz salmon fillets, cut into 1-inch thick slices

2 garlic cloves, crushed

1 cup cherry tomatoes, halved

2 cups Iceberg lettuce, torn

1 tbsp fresh basil, finely chopped

2 tbsp extra-virgin olive oil

2 tbsp Parmesan cheese, grated

1 tbsp white wine vinegar

½ tsp dried thyme, ground

Salt and pepper to taste

Preparation:

Rinse the salmon fillet under running water and pat-dry with a kitchen paper. Transfer to a cutting board and cut into 1-inch thick slices. Set aside.

Bring 2 cups of water to a boil in a deep pot. Place the salmon slices in a steam basket and sprinkle with some salt and thyme. Place the basket on top of the pot and cook for 10 minutes, or until set. Remove the basket from the pot and transfer the salmon to a plate. Cover with aluminum foil and set aside.

In a small mixing bowl, combine garlic, basil, olive oil, cheese, white wine vinegar, salt, and pepper. Mix until combined and set aside.

Rinse the lettuce under running water and drain. Torn into small pieces and place in a salad bowl. Add tomatoes and drizzle all with the previously prepared dressing. Toss to combine and top with salmon slices.

Serve immediately.

Nutritional information per serving: Kcal: 308, Protein: 22.3g, Carbs: 6.9g, Fats: 22.6g

14.   Greek Skewer Salad with Marinated Feta

Ingredients:

1 cup Feta cheese, cut into bite-sized cubes

1 cup cherry tomatoes, whole

1 small cucumber, cut into bite-sized chunks

¼ cup black olives, pitted

1 garlic clove, minced

1 tbsp lime juice, freshly squeezed

2 tbsp olive oil

1 tsp fresh dill, finely chopped

1 tbsp fresh parsley, finely chopped

Salt and pepper

Preparation:

First, prepare the marinade for the Feta cheese. In a mixing bowl, combine olive oil, dill, parsley, lime juice, salt, and pepper. Mix until combined and add Feta cheese. Mix until all the cheese cubes are evenly coated. Refrigerate for 20 minutes.

Wash and prepare the vegetables.

Now, assemble the skewers. Layer cherry tomatoes, olives, cucumber, and marinated Feta cheese. Repeat the process with the remaining ingredients.

Serve immediately.

Nutritional information per serving: Kcal: 254, Protein: 8.6g, Carbs: 9.3g, Fats: 21.4g

15.   Chicken Wrap Salad with Pecans

Ingredients:

4 oz chicken breast, skinless and boneless

½ cup Greek yogurt

1 tsp Dijon mustard

½ whole lemon, juiced

1 tbsp fresh dill, finely chopped

½ cup green grapes

¼ cup toasted pecans

½ cup spring onions, chopped

1 Romaine lettuce head

½ tsp Italian seasoning

Salt and pepper

Preparation:

In a mixing bowl, combine Greek yogurt, Dijon mustard, lemon juice, dill, salt, and pepper. Mix until combined and set aside.

Rinse the chicken under running water and pat-dry with a

kitchen paper. Transfer to a cutting board and cut into bite-sized pieces.

Preheat the oil in a saucepan over medium-high heat. Add chicken and sprinkle with Italian seasoning and salt. Cook for 5 minutes, or until golden brown. Remove from the heat and add to the bowl yogurt mixture.

Add all the remaining ingredients and mix until combined.

Spoon the mixture onto lettuce leaves and wrap. Secure the wraps with a toothpick and serve immediately.

Nutritional information per serving: Kcal: 169, Protein: 19g, Carbs: 14g, Fats: 4.6g

16.   Kale Quinoa Salad with Sesame

Ingredients:

½ cup red quinoa

3 cups fresh kale, chopped

1 small purple onion, chopped

1 tbsp sesame seeds, toasted

¼ cup fresh cilantro, chopped

1 tbsp sesame oil

1 tbsp red wine vinegar

2 tbsp extra-virgin olive oil

Salt and pepper

Preparation:

Rinse the quinoa under running water and drain using a large colander. Place in a deep pot and add 1 cup of water. Bring to a boil over medium-high heat. Reduce the heat to low and simmer for 10-12 minutes, or until all the liquid has been absorbed. Fluff with a fork and set aside.

Place the kale in a colander and rinse thoroughly under running water. Drain and chop into small pieces.

In a large salad bowl, combine quinoa, kale, and onion.

In a small bowl, combine sesame oil, red wine vinegar, olive oil, salt, and pepper. Mix until well combined and drizzle over previously prepared salad. Toss to combine and sprinkle with toasted sesame seeds just before the serving.

Enjoy!

Nutritional information per serving: Kcal: 285, Protein: 6.8g, Carbs: 28.2g, Fats: 17.1g

17.   Orecchiette Salad with Basil

Ingredients:

8 oz orecchiette pasta

1 tbsp fresh basil, finely chopped

2 tbsp sour cream

2 tbsp Feta cheese, crumbled

½ tsp dried rosemary, ground

2 tbsp olive oil

½ tsp dried oregano, ground

Salt and pepper

Preparation:

Place the pasta in deep pot and add water enough to cover. Bring to a boil over medium-high heat. Sprinkle with some salt and cook for 10-12 minutes, or until set. Remove from the heat and drain well. Rinse under cold running water and set aside.

In a food processor, combine fresh basil, sour cream, Feta cheese, rosemary, olive oil, oregano, salt, and pepper. Pulse until smooth.

Transfer the pasta to a salad bowl and drizzle with previously blended sauce mixture. Garnish with some basil and serve immediately.

Enjoy!

Nutritional information per serving: Kcal: 385, Protein: 10.7g, Carbs: 56.3g, Fats: 13.8g

18.   Green Beans Salad with Eggs

Ingredients:

6 oz green beans, chopped

1 large egg, hard-boiled

1 cup cherry tomatoes, chopped

2 cups Romaine lettuce, chopped

¼ cup green olives

1 tbsp Parmesan cheese

1 tsp Dijon mustard

2 tbsp olive oil

2 tsp white wine vinegar

Salt and pepper to taste

Preparation:

Pour 3 cups of water in a saucepan and bring to a boil over medium-high heat. Add chopped green beans and cook for 2 minutes. Remove from the heat and rinse under cold running water immediately. Transfer to a paper-towel lined plate and pat-dry.

Now, place egg in the pot and water enough to cover. Bring to a boil and cook for 10 minutes. Remove from the heat and transfer to the prepared ice cold water bath. When chilled, peel and cut into slices. Set aside.

In a mixing bowl, combine Dijon mustard, olive oil, white wine vinegar, salt, and pepper. Mix until well incorporated and set aside.

Wash and prepare the remaining ingredients.

Combined beans, eggs, tomatoes, and lettuce in a salad bowl. Drizzle with previously prepared dressing and toss to combine. Finally, sprinkle with parmesan cheese.

Enjoy!

Nutritional information per serving: Kcal: 235, Protein: 6.3g, Carbs: 13.3g, Fats: 19.1g

19.   Mackerel Salad

Ingredients:

4 oz mackerel fillets, skinless and boneless

2 cups Iceberg lettuce, chopped

1 medium-sized cucumber, sliced

1 whole lemon, juiced

1 garlic clove, minced

¼ cup sour cream

½ tsp dried thyme, ground

½ tsp dried rosemary, ground

1 tsp Dijon mustard

Salt and pepper

Preparation:

Rinse the fish fillets under running water and pat dry with a kitchen paper. Transfer to a cutting board and cut into small chunks. Sprinkle with some salt and set aside.

Pour 2 cups of water in a deep pot. Bring to a boil over high heat. Place the fish in a steam basket and place on top of the pot. Make sure that the fish doesn't touch the water. Steam until tender and flaky. Remove from the heat and set aside.

In a food processor, combine lemon juice, garlic clove, sour cream, thyme, rosemary, Dijon mustard, salt, and pepper. Pulse until smooth. Set aside.

In a salad bowl, combine lettuce and cucumber. Top with fish and drizzle with previously prepared sauce.

Serve immediately.

Nutritional information per serving: Kcal: 246, Protein: 15.9g, Carbs: 9.3g, Fats: 16.6g

20.   Steak Salad with Caramelized Onions

Ingredients:

1 lb veal steak, cut into thin strips

1 large red onion, sliced

1 tbsp balsamic vinegar

2 tbsp olive oil

2 cups baby arugula, chopped

½ cup plum tomatoes, chopped

½ tsp dried oregano, ground

½ tsp dried thyme, ground

Salt and pepper

Preparation:

Rinse the meat under running water and pat-dry with a kitchen paper. Rub with some salt and pepper and set aside.

In a small saucepan, add balsamic vinegar and 1 tablespoon of olive oil. Heat up over medium-high heat. Add onions and cook for 5 minutes, stirring occasionally. Remove the onions to a plate and add steak. Cook for 3 minutes on each side for medium-rare. Transfer to a cutting board and cut into thin strips. Set aside.

Wash and prepare the remaining ingredients.

In a mixing bowl, combine the remaining olive oil, oregano, thyme, salt, and pepper. Mix until combined.

In a salad bowl, combine baby arugula and plum tomatoes. Drizzle with previously prepared dressing. Toss to combine and then top with steak strips. Top all with caramelized onion mixture and serve immedaitely.

Nutritional information per serving: Kcal: 283, Protein: 30.8g, Carbs: 5.3g, Fats: 15.1g

21.   Steak Salad with Caramelized Onions

Ingredients:

1 lb veal steak, cut into thin strips

1 large red onion, sliced

1 tbsp balsamic vinegar

2 tbsp olive oil

2 cups baby arugula, chopped

½ cup plum tomatoes, chopped

½ tsp dried oregano, ground

½ tsp dried thyme, ground

Salt and pepper

Preparation:

Rinse the meat under running water and pat-dry with a kitchen paper. Rub with some salt and pepper and set aside.

In a small saucepan, add balsamic vinegar and 1 tablespoon of olive oil. Heat up over medium-high heat. Add onions and cook for 5 minutes, stirring occasionally. Remove the onions to a plate and add steak. Cook for 3 minutes on each side for medium-rare. Transfer to a cutting board and cut into thin strips. Set aside.

Wash and prepare the remaining ingredients.

In a mixing bowl, combine the remaining olive oil, oregano, thyme, salt, and pepper. Mix until combined.

In a salad bowl, combine baby arugula and plum tomatoes. Drizzle with previously prepared dressing. Toss to combine and then top with steak strips. Top all with caramelized onion mixture and serve immedaitely.

Nutritional information per serving: Kcal: 283, Protein: 30.8g, Carbs: 5.3g, Fats: 15.1g

22.   Shrimp Avocado Salad with Mango

Ingredients:

10 oz shrimps, cleaned and deveined

1 ripe avocado, sliced

1 ripe mango, chopped

1 whole lime, juiced

2 cups fresh arugula, torn

1 small purple onion, diced

2 tbsp extra-virgin olive oil

¼ tsp cumin powder

Salt and pepper

Preparation:

Pour 2 cups of water in a deep pot. Bring to a boil over medium-high heat. Place the shrimps in a steam basket and sprinkle with some salt. Place the basket on top of the pot and cook for 5-8 minutes. Remove the basket from the pot and set aside.

In a small bowl, combine olive oil, lime juice, cumin powder, and salt. Mix until combined and set aside.

Wash and prepare all the remaining fruit and vegetables.

Now, combine arugula, avocado, mango, and onion in a large salad bowl. Drizzle with previously prepared dressing and toss to combine. Top with shrimps and serve immediately.

Enjoy!

Nutritional information per serving: Kcal: 307, Protein: 18.3g, Carbs: 20g, Fats: 18.4g

23.   Chickpea Tomato Salad with Spinach

Ingredients:

1 cup canned chickpeas, drained and rinsed

1 large cucumber, chopped

2 cups cherry tomatoes, chopped

½ ripe avocado, chopped

2 oz Feta cheese, crumbled

2 tbsp fresh parsley, finely chopped

2 tbsp extra -virgin olive oil

½ whole lemon, freshly juiced

1 tsp Dijon mustard

2 garlic cloves, minced

1 tbsp fresh basil, finely chopped

½ tsp dried oregano, ground

Salt

Preparation:

Place the chickpeas in a colander and rinse well under cold

running water. Drain well and transfer to a large salad bowl. Set aside.

Rinse the cherry tomatoes and remove the stems. Cut into bite-sized pieces and set aside.

Wash the cucumber and cut into small pieces. Set aside.

In a small mixing bowl, combine olive oil, lemon juice, Dijon mustar, garlic, basil, oregano, and salt. Mix until well combined.

Now, add tomatoes, cucumber, avocado, and cheese to the salad bowl. Drizzle all with previously prepared dressing and toss to combine.

Serve immediately.

Nutritional information per serving: Kcal: 254, Protein: 7.1g, Carbs: 24.1g, Fats: 16g

24.   Creamy Cucumber Garlic Salad

Ingredients:

2 cups Greek yogurt

2 tbsp sour cream

1 large cucumber, finely chopped

2 garlic cloves, minced

½ tsp onion powder

2 tbsp olive oil

½ tsp dried thyme, ground

½ tsp dried rosemary, ground

½ tsp red pepper flakes

Salt

Preparation:

Wash the cucumber and cut into tiny pieces. Set aside.

In a food processor, combine garlic cloves, onion powder, dried thyme, rosemary, red pepper flakes, and salt. Pulse until smooth. Now, gradually add olive oil and pulse until all well incorporated.

In a large bowl, combine Greek yogurt and sour cream. Mix and add garlic mixture. Toss to combine and fill small serving bowls.

Refrigerate for 20 minutes before serving. Optionally, sprinkle with some finely chopped parsley.

Nutritional information per serving: Kcal: 328, Protein: 21.8g, Carbs: 15.9g, Fats: 20.8g

25.   Spicy Tortilla Salad

Ingredients:

½ ripe avocado, chopped

1 large cucumber

1 medium-sized red bell pepper

1 Iceberg lettuce head, chopped

¼ cup canned black beans, drained and rinsed

½ cup Mozzarella cheese, sliced

1 whole wheat tortilla, chopped into bite-sized pieces

2 tbsp olive oil

1 whole lemon, juiced

½ tsp chili powder

¼ tsp smoked paprika, ground

½ tsp salt

½ tsp black pepper, ground

Preparation:

Wash the cucumber and cut lengthwise in half. Using a

teaspoon, scrape out the seeds from each half. Cut into thin slices and set aside.

Peel the avocado and cut in half. Remove the pit and cut into bite-sized pieces and set aside.

In a small bowl, combine olive oil, lemon, juice, chili powder, smoked paprika, salt, and pepper. Mix until combined and set aside.

Now, combine avocado, cucumber, black beans, lettuce, red bell pepper, tortilla, and cheese in a salad bowl. Drizzle with previously prepared dressing and toss to combine.

Serve immediately.

Nutritional information per serving: Kcal: 299, Protein: 8.5g, Carbs: 30.9g, Fats: 17.8g

26.　Swiss Cheese Kale Salad with Eggs

Ingredients:

¼ cup Swiss cheese, thinly sliced

2 cups fresh kale, torn

1 large egg, hard-boiled

1 shallot, finely chopped

1 tsp Dijon mustard

½ tsp garlic powder

1 tbsp chives, finely chopped

Salt and pepper to taste

Preparation:

Place the eggs in a deep pot. Add water enough to cover and bring to a boil over medium-high heat. Cook for 10-12 minutes and remove from the heat. Drain and transfer to a bowl with ice cold water. Add a few ice cubes and let it sit for 5 minutes to chill. Peel and cut into thin wedges. Set aside.

Using a large colander, rinse the kale under running water and drain. Torn into small pieces and set aside.

In a small bowl, combine shallot, Dijon mustard, garlic, chives, salt, and pepper. Mix until combined and set aside.

In a large salad bowl, combine kale, eggs, and Swiss cheese. Drizzle with previously prepared dressing and toss to combine.

Serve immediately.

Nutritional information per serving: Kcal: 256, Protein: 18.4g, Carbs: 18.9g, Fats: 12.7g

27.   Shrimp Taco Salad

Ingredients:

10 oz shrimps, cleaned and deveined

1 cup cherry tomatoes, halved

2 cups Romaine lettuce, chopped

2 tbsp corn kernels

1 tbsp olive oil

2 tbsp fresh cilantro, finely chopped

1 whole lime, juiced

1 tsp honey

½ tsp cumin powder

½ tsp smoked paprika

¼ tsp black pepper, ground

Salt

Preparation:

Pour 2 cups of water in a deep pot. Bring it to a boil over medium-high heat. Place the shrimps in a steam basket and put on top of the pot. Cook for 10 minutes. Remove the basket from the pot and set aside.

In a small mixing bowl, combine olive oil, lime juice, honey, cumin powder, smoked paprika, pepper, and salt. Mix until combined and set aside.

In a large mixing bowl, combine cherry tomatoes, lettuce, and corn. Top with shrimps and drizzle with previously prepared dressing. Toss to combine and sprinkle all with fresh cilantro before serving.

Enjoy!

Nutritional information per serving: Kcal: 256, Protein: 18.4g, Carbs: 18.9g, Fats: 12.7g

28.   Ginger Salmon Salad

Ingredients:

6 oz smoked salmon, cut into thin slices

2 tsp fresh ginger, shredded

1 tbsp soy sauce

1 garlic clove, minced

1 tbsp sesame seeds

2 tbsp olive oil

1 tbsp white wine vinegar

2 cups baby spinach

1 large carrot, shredded

2 tbsp spring onions, chopped

½ tsp dried thyme, ground

Salt and pepper

Preparation:

In a small mixing bowl, combine ginger, soy sauce, garlic, sesame seeds, olive oil, white wine vinegar, thyme, salt, and pepper. Mix until well combined and set aside.

Place the spinach in a large colander. Rinse under running water and drain. Cut into bite-sized pieces and set aside.

Now, place the spinach on the bottom of your serving bowl and top with smoked salmon slices. Drizzle with previously prepared dressing and serve immediately.

Enjoy!

Nutritional information per serving: Kcal: 284, Protein: 18.4g, Carbs: 8.7g, Fats: 20.2g

29.   Fusilli Salad with Balsamic Glaze

Ingredients:

10 oz fusilli pasta

1 cup cherry tomatoes

1 large yellow bell pepper, chopped

1 onion, sliced

2 tbsp extra-virgin olive oil

1 tbsp balsamic vinegar

1 garlic clove, crushed

½ tsp Italian seasoning

Salt and pepper

Preparation:

Place the pasta in a deep pot and add water enough water to cover. Sprinkle with some salt and bring to a boil over medium-high heat. Cook for 10-12 minutes. Remove from the heat and drain well. Transfer to a large colander and rinse under cold running water. Set aside.

In a small mixing bowl, combine olive oil balsamic vinegar, garlic, Italian seasoning, salt, and pepper. Mix until well combined.

In a large salad bowl, combine pasta, cherry tomatoes, yellow bell pepper, and onion. Drizzle all with previously prepared glaze and toss to combine.

Serve cold.

Nutritional information per serving: Kcal: 342, Protein: 10.2g, Carbs: 59.4g, Fats: 8.2g

30.   Spicy Rice Taco Salad

Ingredients:

½ cup brown rice

½ cup tomatoes, chopped

1/4 cup canned black beans

½ ripe avocado, sliced

2 tbsp fresh cilantro, finely chopped

½ cup Cheddar cheese, shredded

1 cup Greek yogurt

2 tbsp olive oil

2 tsp honey

1 tbsp apple cider vinegar

1 whole lime, freshly juiced

½ Jalapeno pepper, diced

1 tsp Taco seasoning

Salt

Preparation:

Place the rice in a deep pot and add ¾ cup of water. Sprinkle with some salt and bring to a boil over medium-high heat. Reduce the heat to low and cook for 10-15 minutes, or until almost all the liquid has been absporbed.

In a mixing bowl, combine Greek yogurt, olive oil, honey, apple cider vinegar, lime juice, diced Jalapeno pepper, Taco seasoning, and salt. Mix until combined and set aside.

In a large salad bowl, combine tomatoes, black beans, and avocado. Drizzle with previously prepared dressing and sprinkle all with fresh cilantro. Optionally, garnish with some lime wedges before serving.

Enjoy!

Nutritional information per serving: Kcal: 313, Protein: 12.9g, Carbs: 26.5g, Fats: 18.2g

31.   Zucchini Noodle Salad

Ingredients:

2 large zucchinis

½ cup Mozzarella cheese, sliced

½ cup cherry tomatoes, halved

1 tbsp fresh basil, finely chopped

1 tbsp balsamic vinegar

2 tbsp extra-virgin olive oil

½ tsp dried thyme, ground

½ tsp dried parsley, ground

Salt and pepper to taste

Preparation:

In a small mixing bowl, combine olive oil, balsamic vinegar, thyme, parsley, salt, and pepper. Mix until combined and set aside.

Wash the zucchinis and remove the top stem. Run through a spiralizer and transfer to a large bowl. Drizzle with previously prepared mixture and toss well. Cover the bowl with a plastic foil and let it marinate for 20 minutes.

Meanwhile, prepare the remaining ingredients.

In a large salad bowl, combine cheese, cherry tomatoes, and marinated zucchinis. Sprinkle all with some salt, pepper, and finely chopped basil leaves.

Serve immediately.

Nutritional information per serving: Kcal: 313, Protein: 12.9g, Carbs: 26.5g, Fats: 18.2g

32.   Gala Spinach Salad

Ingredients:

2 cups fresh baby spinach

1 Gala apple, thinly sliced

¼ cup Feta cheese, crumbled

1 small purple onion, sliced

2 tbsp toasted almonds, sliced

2 tbsp olive oil

1 tbsp red wine vinegar

1 garlic clove, minced

1 tsp Dijon mustard

Salt and pepper to taste

Preparation:

Using a large colander, rinse the spinach under running water. Drain and chop into small pieces. Set aside.

Wash the apple and cut in half. Remove the core and cut into bite-sized pieces. Set aside.

In a small mixing bowl, combine olive oil, red wine vinegar, garlic, Dijon mustard, salt, and pepper. Mix until combined and set aside.

Now, in a large salad bowl, combine spinach, apple, cheese, and onion. Drizzle all with previously prepared dressing and top with toasted almonds before serving.

You can change the red wine vinegar with lemon or lime juice. However, it is completely optional.

Enjoy!

Nutritional information per serving: Kcal: 265, Protein: 5.5g, Carbs: 15.1g, Fats: 21.5g

33.   Creamy Tuna Salad

Ingredients:

½ cup canned tuna, drained

1 small purple onion, diced

2 tbsp fresh parsley, finely chopped

2 tbsp corn, drained and rinsed

¼ cup black olives, pitted

1 small cucumber, diced

2 tbsp Greek yogurt

2 tbsp olive oil

½ tsp smoked paprika

Salt and pepper to taste

Preparation:

In a small mixing bowl, combine Greek yogurt, olive oil, smoked paprika, salt, and pepper. Mix until combined and set aside.

Rinse the corn under running water and drain. Set aside.

Peel the onion and finely chop into small pieces. Set aside.

Wash the cucumber and dice into small pieces. Set aside.

Place the tuna in a siever and rinse under running water. Drain by pressing with a spoon. Transfer to a salad bowl and add finely chopped parsley, corn, and diced onion. Mix once and then drizzle with previously prepared dressing. Toss until well combined.

Optionally, spoon the mixture onto a lettuce leaves and serve.

Nutritional information per serving: Kcal: 267, Protein: 13g, Carbs: 26.5g, Fats: 14.5g

34.   Stuffed Avocado Salad

Ingredients:

1 ripe avocado, halved

4 medium-sized shrimps, cleaned and deveined

¼ cup cherry tomatoes, chopped

1 tbsp canned corn, drained and rinsed

½ tsp dried rosemary, ground

¼ tsp dried thyme, ground

½ whole lemon, juiced

1 tbsp olive oil

¼ tsp black pepper, ground

¼ tsp sea salt

Preparation:

Cut the avocado into halves and remove the pit. Gently scoop out the inner flesh, leaving a thin layer on the sides. Set aside.

Pour 2 cups of water in a deep pot. Bring to a boil over medium-high heat. Meanwhile, place the shrimps into the steam basket. Place the basket on top of the pot and steam for 10 minutes, or until pink. Remove from the heat and set aside.

In a mixing bowl, combine cherry tomatoes, corn, rosemary, thyme, lemon juice, olive oil, pepper, and salt. Mix until combined and add shrimps. Mix again until all well incorporated.

Spoon the mixture into prepared avocado shells. Optionally, garnish with some fresh basil.

You can use the scooped avocado flesh and mix it into the salad. However, it's optional.

Enjoy!

Nutritional information per serving: Kcal: 389, Protein: 14.7g, Carbs: 25.1g, Fats: 28.4g

35.   Strawberry Spinach Salad with Quinoa

Ingredients:

¼ cup white quinoa

2 cups strawberries, chopped

2 cups fresh spinach, torn

¼ cup Feta cheese, crumbled

2 tbsp toasted almonds

2 tbsp olive oil

1 tbsp balsamic vinegar

½ tsp dried parsley, ground

¼ tsp dried oregano, ground

Salt and pepper

Preparation:

Place the quinoa in a heavy-bottomed pot and add ½ cup of water. Bring to a boil over medium-high heat. Reduce the heat to low and simmer for 10-15 minutes. Remove from the heat and fluff with a fork. Set aside.

Rinse the strawberries using a large colander. Remove the

stems and chop into bite-sized pieces. Set aside.

Rinse the spinach under running water and drain. Chop into small pieces and set aside.

In a small mixing bowl, combine olive oil, balsamic vinegar, parsley, oregano, salt, and pepper. Mix until well combined and set aside.

In a large salad bowl, add quinoa, strawberries, spinach, and cheese. Drizzle with previously prepared dressing and toss to combine. Finally, top with toasted almonds and serve immediately.

Nutritional information per serving: Kcal: 337, Protein: 8.8g, Carbs: 28.1g, Fats: 22.8g

36.   Skirt Steak Salad with Peaches

Ingredients:

6 oz lean skirt steak

2 cups fresh arugula, chopped

1 large peach, thinly sliced

¼ cup Feta cheese, chopped

1 garlic clove, minced

1 tbsp olive oil

2 tbsp balsamic vinegar

½ tsp salt

¼ tsp black pepper, ground

¼ tsp dried thyme, ground

1 whole lemon, juiced

Preparation:

In a small mixing bowl, combine garlic, 1 tablespoon of balsamic vinegar, and salt. Mix until combined. Brush the steak with this mixture and let it sit for 15 minutes on room temperature. This will allow the juices to penetrate into the meat.

Preheat the grill to high heat. Generously brush the meat with olive oil and grill for 3 minutes on each side for medium-rare. Remove from the grill and cut into thin slices. Set aside.

Combine lemon juice, the remaining balsamic vinegar, salt, pepper, and thyme in a small bowl. Mix until combined and set aside.

Rinse the arugula under running water. Drain and chop into small pieces. Transfer to a large salad bowl along with peach and cheese. Top with steak slices and drizzle all with previously prepared dressing.

Serve immediately.

Nutritional information per serving: Kcal: 325, Protein: 26.7g, Carbs: 9.4g, Fats: 19.9g

37.   Kiwi Mango Salad with Chia

Ingredients:

3 whole kiwis, peeled

1 ripe mango, chopped

1 small Granny Smith's apple, cored

1 large orange, peeled

1 cup green grapes

½ cup fresh blueberries

½ cup fresh raspberries

1 cup fresh strawberries

2 tbsp lime juice, freshly squeezed

1 tbsp honey

1 tbsp chia seeds

Preparation:

Peel the kiwis and cut into thin rings. Set aside.

Wash the mango and cut in half, avoiding the pit in the middle. Holding mango vertically, trim off the remaining flesh of the pit. Peel the skin and cut into small chunks. Set aside.

Wash the apple and cut lengthwise in half. Remove the core and cut into bite-sized pieces.

In a large colander, combine grapes, blueberries, raspberries, and strawberries. Rinse under running water and drain. Remove the stems from grapes and strawberries, if any. Chop the strawberries into small pieces and set aside.

In a small mixing bowl, combine lime juice, honey, and chia seeds. Mix until combined and set aside.

In a large bowl, combine all the fruit and drizzle with the dressing. Toss to combine and refrigerate for 20 minutes before serving.

Enjoy!

Nutritional information per serving: Kcal: 290, Protein: 4.6g, Carbs: 69.6g, Fats: 3g

38.   Avocado Shrimp Salad

Ingredients:

1 ripe avocado, chunked

6 oz fresh shrimps, cleaned and deveined

1 small Jalapeno pepper, finely chopped

1 garlic clove, minced

2 tbsp lime juice, freshly squeezed

1 tbsp fresh cilantro, finely chopped

2 tbsp olive oil

¼ tsp dried thyme, ground

½ tsp smoked paprika, ground

Salt and pepper to taste

Preparation:

Cut the avocado lengthwise in half. Remove the pit and cut into bite-sized chunks. Set aside.

Pour 2 cups of water in a deep pot. Bring to a boil over medium-high heat. Place the shrimps in a steam basket and place on top of the pot. Steam for 3 minutes and gently toss. Continue to steam for another 3 minutes. Remove from the heat and set aside.

In a small mixing bowl, combine jalapeno pepper, garlic, lime juice, olive oil, thyme, smoked paprika, salt, and pepper to taste. Mix until combined.

In a large salad bowl, combine avocado and shrimps. Drizzle with previously prepared dressing and toss to combine.

Serve immediately.

Nutritional information per serving: Kcal: 292, Protein: 14.4g, Carbs: 8.7g, Fats: 23.5g

39.   Spinach Orzo Salad

Ingredients:

3 cups fresh spinach, chopped

½ cup orzo pasta

1 cup cherry tomatoes, chopped

1 large egg, hard-boiled

1 tbsp olive oil

1 tbsp lemon juice, freshly sqeezed

½ tsp Italian seasoning

¼ cup Feta cheese, crumbled

¼ tsp red pepper flakes

Preparation:

Using a large colander, rinse the spinach under running water. Remove the hard stems and chop into small pieces.

Pour 1 cup of water in a deep pot and bring to a boil over medium-high heat. Place the spinach in a steam basket and sprinkle with some salt. Steam for 3 minutes. Remove from the heat and set aside.

Place the pasta in a deep pot and cover with water. Bring to a boil over medium-high heat. Cook for 10 minutes and remove from the heat. Transfer to a colander and rinse under cold water. Set aside.

Place the egg in the pot and add water enough to cover. Bring to a boil over medium-high heat and cook for 10-12 minutes. Remove from the heat and transfer to a prepared ice cold water bath. Let it chill for 2-3 minutes and then peel. Cut into thin wedges and set aside.

In a small mixing bowl, combine, olive oil, lemon juice, Italian seasoning, and red pepper flakes. Mix until combined and set aside.

In a large salad bowl, combine spinach, orzo, cheese, cherry tomatoes, and egg. Drizzle all with previously prepared dressing and serve.

Nutritional information per serving: Kcal: 252, Protein: 10.5g, Carbs: 22.1g, Fats: 14.5g

40.   Grilled Mushroom Salad with Greens

Ingredients:

1 cup button mushrooms, chopped

1 cup fresh kale, chopped

1 cup fresh broccoli, chopped

2 tbsp bean sprouts

1 large Roma tomato, chopped

1 tbsp olive oil

¼ tsp dried parsley, ground

¼ tsp black pepper, ground

½ tbsp red wine vinegar

Salt

Preparation:

Rinse well the mushrooms and place on a large pieces of paper towel. Wrap and pat-dry. Sprinkle with some salt and set aside.

Preheat the grill to medium-high. Brush the mushrooms with olive oil and place on a rack. Grill for 3-5 minutes, turning occasionally. Remove from the grill and set aside.

In a large colander, combine kale and broccoli. Rinse under running water and drain. Chop into bite-sized pieces and place in a steam basket. Pour 1 cup of water in a deep pot and bring to a boil. Place the basket on top of the pot and steam for 3 minutes. Remove from the pot and set aside.

In a small mixing bowl, combine red wine vinegar, salt, and pepper. Mix until combined and set aside.

In a large salad bowl, combine mushrooms, kale, broccoli, and tomato. Drizzle with previously prepared dressing and top with bean sprouts. Optionally, drizzle with some more olive oil before serving.

Enjoy!

Nutritional information per serving: Kcal: 249, Protein: 9.8g, Carbs: 25.7g, Fats: 15.1g

41.   Swiss Chard Salad with Cashew Sauce

Ingredients:

2 cups Swiss chard, chopped

1 small red bell pepper, chopped

½ cup red cabbage, shredded

1 small purple onion, sliced

½ cup cashews

½ tsp Dijon mustard

1 tsp honey

1 whole lime, freshly juiced

Salt

Preparation:

In a small mixing bowl, combine cashews, Dijon mustard, honey, lime, and a pinch of salt. Add about ½ cup of water and let it sit for 10 minutes.

Meanwhile, place the Swiss chard into a large colander and rinse under running water. Drain and chop into small pieces.

Wash and prepare the remaining vegetables.

Now, transfer the cashew mixture to a food processor and pulse until smooth and creamy.

In a large salad bowl, combine Swiss chard, red bell pepper, red cabbage, and onion. Drizzle all with previously prepared cashew sauce and stir until well coated.

Optionally, garnish with some fresh, finely chopped parsley.

Nutritional information per serving: Kcal: 292, Protein: 7.2g, Carbs: 34.3g, Fats: 16.2g

42. **Spicy Mixed Salad**

Ingredients:

1 large cucumber, sliced

1 cup cherry tomatoes, chopped

1 large yellow bell pepper, chopped

1 cup fresh spinach, chopped

1 tbsp extra-virgin olive oil

1 tbsp flaxseed oil

1 tsp apple cider vinegar

½ tsp dried oregano, ground

¼ tsp garlic powder

¼ tsp curry powder

¼ tsp cayenne pepper

Salt

Preparation:

Wash the cucumber and cut into thick slices. Set aside.

Rinse the tomatoes and remove the stems. Cut into bite-sized pieces and set aside.

Wash the bell pepper and cut lengthwise in half. Remove the stem and seeds. Chop into small pieces and set aside.

Rinse the spinach under running water using a large colander. Drain and chop into small pieces. Set aside.

In a small mixing bowl, combine olive oil, flaxseed oil, apple cider vinegar, dried oregano, garlic powder, curry powder, cayenne pepper, and a pinch of salt. Mix until combined and set aside.

In a large salad bowl, combine cucumber, tomatoes, bell pepper, and spinach. Drizzle with previously prepared dressing and toss to combine.

Optionally, add some crumbled Feta cheese for an extra flavor.

Nutritional information per serving: Kcal: 191, Protein: 3g, Carbs: 14.8g, Fats: 14.7g

43.   Chickpea Salad with Sumac Dressing

Ingredients:

½ cup chickpeas, soaked overnight

1 large tomato, chopped

1 small purple onion, diced

2 tbsp cottage cheese, crumbled

1 tbsp Italian parsley, finely chopped

¼ cup olives, pitted

1 garlic clove, crushed

2 tbsp extra-virgin olive oil

½ whole lime, juiced

1 tbsp scallions, chopped

1 tsp sumac

¼ tsp cumin powder

½ tsp smoked paprika, ground

¼ tsp red pepper flakes

Salt and pepper to taste

2 cups Romaine lettuce, roughly chopped

Preparation:

Drain and rinse the soaked chickpeas. Transfer to a deep pot and 1-1 ½ cup of water. Bring to a boil over medium-high heat. Reduce the heat to low and cook for about 45 minutes to 1 hour. If needed, add more water while cooking. When done, remove from the heat and drain. Set aside.

In a small mixing bowl, combine garlic, olive oil, lime juice, sumac, cumin powder, smoked paprika, red pepper flakes, salt, and pepper. Mix until well incorporated and set aside.

In a large salad bowl, combine cooked chickpeas,tomato, onion, cottage cheese, olives, and parsley. Drizzle all with previously prepared dressing and toss to combine. Refrigerate for 30 minutes.

Now, spread the lettuce over the serving plate and spoon the salad on top.

Serve immediately.

Nutritional information per serving: Kcal: 332, Protein: 11.2g, Carbs: 33.9g, Fats: 18.7g

44. Grapefruit Arugula Salad

Ingredients:

3 grapefruits, peeled and wedged

3 cups fresh arugula, chopped

½ ripe avocado, chopped

1 tbsp sunflower seeds

1 tbsp almonds, chopped

2 tbsp avocado oil

1 tbsp white wine vinegar

1 whole lime, freshly juiced

1 tsp yellow mustard

1 tsp turmeric powder

1 tbsp nutritional yeast

Salt and pepper

Preparation:

In a small mixing bowl, combine avocado oil, white wine vinegar, lime juice, yellow mustard, turmeric powder, nutritional yeast, salt, and pepper. Mix until all well incorporated and set aside.

Place the arugula in a large colander and rinse under running water. Drain and chop into small pieces. Set aside.

Peel the grapefruits and divide into wedges. Cut each wedge in half and set aside.

Peel the avocado and cut lengthwise in half. Remove the pit and chop one half into bite-sized pieces. Reserve the rest in the refrigerator.

In a large salad bowl, combine arugula, grapefruit, and avocado. Drizzle all with previously prepared dressing and serve immediately.

Enjoy!

Nutritional information per serving: Kcal: 284, Protein: 6.4g, Carbs: 25.1g, Fats: 19.9g

45.   Hokkaido Salad

Ingredients:

2 cups hokkaido pumpkin, cubed

2 cups fresh kale, chopped

½ cup Feta cheese, cubed

1 small onion, diced

1 garlic clove, minced

1 tbsp pumpkin seeds

1 tbsp avocado oil

1 tbsp hard goat's cheese, grated

Salt and pepper

Preparation:

Preheat the oven to 350 degrees. Line some parchment paper over a large baking sheet and set aside.

Cut the pumpkin in half and scoop out the seeds. Cut and peel 2 large wedges. Chop into bite-sized cubes and fill the measuring cup. Reserve the rest in the refrigerator. Spread the pumpkin over the prepared sheet and sprinkle with olive oil, salt, and pepper. Place it in the oven and roast for

20 minutes.

Meanwhile, prepare the remaining ingredients.

Rinse the kale under running water. Drain and remove the hard ribs. Chop into small pieces and set aside.

In a food processor, combine avocado oil, garlic, onion, pumpkin seeds, salt, and pepper. Pulse until smooth and well incorporated.

In a large salad bowl, combine pumpkin, kale, and cheese. Drizzle with previously prepared dressing and toss to combine.

Serve cold.

Nutritional information per serving: Kcal: 278, Protein: 12.6g, Carbs: 33.3g, Fats: 12.8g

46.   Quinoa Bean Salad with Mango

Ingredients:

½ cup canned black beans, drained and rinsed

½ cup quinoa

1 ripe mango, chopped

1 small red bell pepper, diced

2 tbsp fresh parsley, finely chopped

½ whole lime, freshly juiced

2 tbsp olive oil

½ tsp black pepper

¼ tsp salt

Preparation:

Place the quinoa in a colander and rinse thoroughly under runnning water. Drain and transfer to a deep pot. Add 1 cup of water and bring to a boil over medium-high heat. Reduce the heat to low and cook for 10-15 minutes, or until all the liquid has been soaked up and evaporated. Stir once and remove from the heat. Set aside.

Rinse and drain the black beans and place in a large salad

bowl along with chopped mango, and bell pepper.

In a small mixing bowl, combine parlsey, lime, olive oil, black pepper, and salt. Mix until combined and drizzle over the salad.

Toss again to combine and serve immediately.

Nutritional information per serving: Kcal: 302, Protein: 7.9g, Carbs: 45g, Fats: 11.7g

47.   Eastern Halloumi Salad with Beluga Lentils

Ingredients:

½ cup halloumi cheese

1 cup beluga lentils, soaked overnight

1 tbsp pine nuts

1 large cucumber, sliced

¼ cup black olives

1 tbsp fresh coriander, finely chopped

1 tbsp wild garlic, finely chopped

1 tbsp dried seaweed, chopped

1 whole lime, freshly juiced

Salt and pepper

Preparation:

Preheat a large saucepan over medium-high heat. Add cheese and fry for 3-4 minutes, or until golden brown and crispy. Remove from the heat and set aside.

Rinse and drain the lentils. Place in a deep bowl and add 2 cups of water. Bring to a boil over medium-high heat. Cook for 30 minutes and remove from the heat. Drain well and set aside.

In a large salad bowl, combine halloumi cheese, lentils, cucumber, and olives. Sprinkle all with lime juice, coriander, wild garlic, seaweed, salt, and pepper. Mix until well combined and top pine nuts before serving.

Nutritional information per serving: Kcal: 260, Protein: 15.2g, Carbs: 18.6g, Fats: 14.8g

48. Roasted Beet Salad with Mixed Greens

Ingredients:

2 medium-sized beets, sliced

1 cup fresh spinach, chopped

1 cup fresh arugula, chopped

1 cup fresh kale, chopped

1 large orange, peeled and wedged

2 tbsp pumpkin seeds

1 whole lime, freshly squeezed

¼ cup pomegranate seeds

1 tsp Italian seasoning

¼ tsp garlic powder

1 tbsp apple cider vinegar

3 tbsp olive oil

Salt and pepper to taste

Preparation:

Preheat the oven to 400 degrees. Line some parchment

paper over a baking sheet and set aside.

Wash the beets and transfer to a cutting board. Using a sharp knife, trim off the green parts and cut into thin slices. Sprinkle with some salt and spread over the prepared baking sheet. Place it in the oven and roast for 35-40 minutes, or until fork-tender. Remove from the oven and set aside.

In a small mixing bowl, combine olive oil, lime juice, Italian seasoning, garlic powder, apple cider vinegar, salt, and pepper. Mix until well combined and set aside.

Combine all greens in a large colander and rinse under running water. Drain well and chop into small pieces.

In a large salad bowl, place the greens and top with beets. Sprinkle all with previously prepared dressing and toss to combine.

Serve immediately.

Nutritional information per serving: Kcal: 239, Protein: 4.4g, Carbs: 20.2g, Fats: 17.4g

49. Sweet Potato Carrot Salad

Ingredients:

1 medium-sized sweet potato, peeled and chunked

1 large carrot, sliced

1 cup asparagus, trimmed and chopped

1 small onion, diced

2 tbsp olive oil

1 tbsp white wine vinegar

1 tsp Dijon mustard

¼ cup Greek yogurt

¼ tsp dried dill, ground

¼ tsp dried rosemary, ground

Salt and pepper

Preparation:

Pour 4 cups of water in a deep pot and bring it to a boil over medium-high heat. Add chopped potatoes and sliced carrot. Cook for 10 minutes.

Meanwhile, rinse and drain the asparagus. Trim of the

woody ends and chop into bite-sized pieces. Add to the pot and continue to cook for 5 more minutes.

Remove from the heat and drain well. Using a large slotted spoon, remove the vegetables to a bowl and let it cool.

In a small mixing bowl, combine olive oil, vinegar, mustard, yogurt, dill, rosemary, salt, and pepper. Mix until smooth and drizzle over the vegetables. Toss to combine and serve immediately.

Nutritional information per serving: Kcal: 225, Protein: 4.5g, Carbs: 22g, Fats: 14.6g

ADDITIONAL TITLES FROM THIS AUTHOR

70 Effective Meal Recipes to Prevent and Solve Being Overweight: Burn Fat Fast by Using Proper Dieting and Smart Nutrition

By Joe Correa CSN

48 Acne Solving Meal Recipes: The Fast and Natural Path to Fixing Your Acne Problems in Less Than 10 Days!

By Joe Correa CSN

41 Alzheimer's Preventing Meal Recipes: Reduce or Eliminate Your Alzheimer's Condition in 30 Days or Less!

By Joe Correa CSN

70 Effective Breast Cancer Meal Recipes: Prevent and Fight Breast Cancer with Smart Nutrition and Powerful Foods

By Joe Correa CSN

CPSIA information can be obtained
at www.ICGtesting.com
Printed in the USA
BVHW081233010419
544230BV00029B/1629/P